JOURNAL BELONGS TO

_____

_____

_____

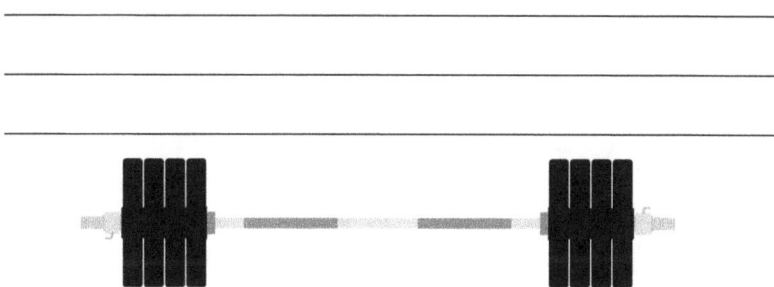

MEASUREMENTS

DATE							
UPPER ARM L							
UPPER ARM R							
FOREARM L							
FOREARM R							
THIGH L							
THIGH R							
CALF L							
CALF R							
WAIST							
CHEST							
SHOULDER							
WEIGHT							

NOTES

MONTH:

SUNDAY	MONDAY	TUESDAY	WEDNESDAY	THURSDAY	FRIDAY	SATURDAY

NOTES

MONTH:

WORKOUT ROUTINE

SUNDAY	MONDAY	TUESDAY	WEDNESDAY	THURSDAY	FRIDAY	SATURDAY

NOTES

MONTH:

SUNDAY	MONDAY	TUESDAY	WEDNESDAY	THURSDAY	FRIDAY	SATURDAY

NOTES

DATE _____

EXERCISE	SETS	1	2	3	4	5	6	7	8	9	10
	WEIGHT										
	REPS										
	WEIGHT										
	REPS										
	WEIGHT										
	REPS										
	WEIGHT										
	REPS										
	WEIGHT										
	REPS										
	WEIGHT										
	REPS										
	WEIGHT										
	REPS										
	WEIGHT										
	REPS										
	WEIGHT										
	REPS										

NOTES–*(Energy levels, thoughts, adjustments needed.)*

DATE _____

BREAKFAST

MACROS	
PROTEIN	%
CARBS	%
FAT	%
CALORIES	

LUNCH

MACROS	
PROTEIN	%
CARBS	%
FAT	%
CALORIES	

DINNER

MACROS	
PROTEIN	%
CARBS	%
FAT	%
CALORIES	

SNACKS

MACROS	
PROTEIN	%
CARBS	%
FAT	%
CALORIES	

SUPPLEMENTS

TOTAL MACROS	
PROTEIN	%
CARBS	%
FAT	%
CALORIES	

NOTES

WATER (12 OZ)

DATE _____

EXERCISE	SETS	1	2	3	4	5	6	7	8	9	10
	WEIGHT										
	REPS										
	WEIGHT										
	REPS										
	WEIGHT										
	REPS										
	WEIGHT										
	REPS										
	WEIGHT										
	REPS										
	WEIGHT										
	REPS										
	WEIGHT										
	REPS										
	WEIGHT										
	REPS										
	WEIGHT										
	REPS										

NOTES–*(Energy levels, thoughts, adjustments needed.)*

DATE _____

BREAKFAST

MACROS	
PROTEIN	%
CARBS	%
FAT	%
CALORIES	

LUNCH

MACROS	
PROTEIN	%
CARBS	%
FAT	%
CALORIES	

DINNER

MACROS	
PROTEIN	%
CARBS	%
FAT	%
CALORIES	

SNACKS

MACROS	
PROTEIN	%
CARBS	%
FAT	%
CALORIES	

SUPPLEMENTS

TOTAL MACROS	
PROTEIN	%
CARBS	%
FAT	%
CALORIES	

NOTES

WATER (12 OZ)

DATE _____

EXERCISE	SETS	1	2	3	4	5	6	7	8	9	10
	WEIGHT										
	REPS										
	WEIGHT										
	REPS										
	WEIGHT										
	REPS										
	WEIGHT										
	REPS										
	WEIGHT										
	REPS										
	WEIGHT										
	REPS										
	WEIGHT										
	REPS										
	WEIGHT										
	REPS										
	WEIGHT										
	REPS										

NOTES–(Energy levels, thoughts, adjustments needed.)

DATE _____

BREAKFAST

MACROS	
PROTEIN	%
CARBS	%
FAT	%
CALORIES	

LUNCH

MACROS	
PROTEIN	%
CARBS	%
FAT	%
CALORIES	

DINNER

MACROS	
PROTEIN	%
CARBS	%
FAT	%
CALORIES	

SNACKS

MACROS	
PROTEIN	%
CARBS	%
FAT	%
CALORIES	

SUPPLEMENTS

TOTAL MACROS	
PROTEIN	%
CARBS	%
FAT	%
CALORIES	

NOTES

WATER (12 OZ)

DATE _____

EXERCISE	SETS	1	2	3	4	5	6	7	8	9	10
	WEIGHT										
	REPS										
	WEIGHT										
	REPS										
	WEIGHT										
	REPS										
	WEIGHT										
	REPS										
	WEIGHT										
	REPS										
	WEIGHT										
	REPS										
	WEIGHT										
	REPS										
	WEIGHT										
	REPS										
	WEIGHT										
	REPS										

NOTES–(Energy levels, thoughts, adjustments needed.)

DATE _____

BREAKFAST

MACROS	
PROTEIN	%
CARBS	%
FAT	%
CALORIES	

LUNCH

MACROS	
PROTEIN	%
CARBS	%
FAT	%
CALORIES	

DINNER

MACROS	
PROTEIN	%
CARBS	%
FAT	%
CALORIES	

SNACKS

MACROS	
PROTEIN	%
CARBS	%
FAT	%
CALORIES	

SUPPLEMENTS

TOTAL MACROS	
PROTEIN	%
CARBS	%
FAT	%
CALORIES	

NOTES

WATER (12 OZ)

DATE _____

EXERCISE	SETS	1	2	3	4	5	6	7	8	9	10
	WEIGHT										
	REPS										
	WEIGHT										
	REPS										
	WEIGHT										
	REPS										
	WEIGHT										
	REPS										
	WEIGHT										
	REPS										
	WEIGHT										
	REPS										
	WEIGHT										
	REPS										
	WEIGHT										
	REPS										
	WEIGHT										
	REPS										

NOTES–(Energy levels, thoughts, adjustments needed.)

DATE _____

BREAKFAST		MACROS	
		PROTEIN	%
		CARBS	%
		FAT	%
		CALORIES	

LUNCH		MACROS	
		PROTEIN	%
		CARBS	%
		FAT	%
		CALORIES	

DINNER		MACROS	
		PROTEIN	%
		CARBS	%
		FAT	%
		CALORIES	

SNACKS		MACROS	
		PROTEIN	%
		CARBS	%
		FAT	%
		CALORIES	

SUPPLEMENTS		TOTAL MACROS	
		PROTEIN	%
		CARBS	%
		FAT	%
		CALORIES	

NOTES

WATER (12 OZ)

DATE _____

EXERCISE	SETS	1	2	3	4	5	6	7	8	9	10
	WEIGHT										
	REPS										
	WEIGHT										
	REPS										
	WEIGHT										
	REPS										
	WEIGHT										
	REPS										
	WEIGHT										
	REPS										
	WEIGHT										
	REPS										
	WEIGHT										
	REPS										
	WEIGHT										
	REPS										
	WEIGHT										
	REPS										

NOTES–*(Energy levels, thoughts, adjustments needed.)*

DATE _____

BREAKFAST

MACROS		
PROTEIN		%
CARBS		%
FAT		%
CALORIES		

LUNCH

MACROS		
PROTEIN		%
CARBS		%
FAT		%
CALORIES		

DINNER

MACROS		
PROTEIN		%
CARBS		%
FAT		%
CALORIES		

SNACKS

MACROS		
PROTEIN		%
CARBS		%
FAT		%
CALORIES		

SUPPLEMENTS

TOTAL MACROS		
PROTEIN		%
CARBS		%
FAT		%
CALORIES		

NOTES

WATER (12 OZ)

DATE _____

EXERCISE	SETS	1	2	3	4	5	6	7	8	9	10
	WEIGHT										
	REPS										
	WEIGHT										
	REPS										
	WEIGHT										
	REPS										
	WEIGHT										
	REPS										
	WEIGHT										
	REPS										
	WEIGHT										
	REPS										
	WEIGHT										
	REPS										
	WEIGHT										
	REPS										
	WEIGHT										
	REPS										

NOTES–(Energy levels, thoughts, adjustments needed.)

DATE _____

BREAKFAST

MACROS	
PROTEIN	%
CARBS	%
FAT	%
CALORIES	

LUNCH

MACROS	
PROTEIN	%
CARBS	%
FAT	%
CALORIES	

DINNER

MACROS	
PROTEIN	%
CARBS	%
FAT	%
CALORIES	

SNACKS

MACROS	
PROTEIN	%
CARBS	%
FAT	%
CALORIES	

SUPPLEMENTS

TOTAL MACROS	
PROTEIN	%
CARBS	%
FAT	%
CALORIES	

NOTES

WATER (12 OZ)

DATE _____

EXERCISE	SETS	1	2	3	4	5	6	7	8	9	10
	WEIGHT										
	REPS										
	WEIGHT										
	REPS										
	WEIGHT										
	REPS										
	WEIGHT										
	REPS										
	WEIGHT										
	REPS										
	WEIGHT										
	REPS										
	WEIGHT										
	REPS										
	WEIGHT										
	REPS										
	WEIGHT										
	REPS										

NOTES–(Energy levels, thoughts, adjustments needed.)

DATE _____

BREAKFAST		MACROS	
		PROTEIN	%
		CARBS	%
		FAT	%
		CALORIES	

LUNCH		MACROS	
		PROTEIN	%
		CARBS	%
		FAT	%
		CALORIES	

DINNER		MACROS	
		PROTEIN	%
		CARBS	%
		FAT	%
		CALORIES	

SNACKS		MACROS	
		PROTEIN	%
		CARBS	%
		FAT	%
		CALORIES	

SUPPLEMENTS		TOTAL MACROS	
		PROTEIN	%
		CARBS	%
		FAT	%
		CALORIES	

NOTES

WATER (12 OZ)

DATE _____

EXERCISE	SETS	1	2	3	4	5	6	7	8	9	10
	WEIGHT										
	REPS										
	WEIGHT										
	REPS										
	WEIGHT										
	REPS										
	WEIGHT										
	REPS										
	WEIGHT										
	REPS										
	WEIGHT										
	REPS										
	WEIGHT										
	REPS										
	WEIGHT										
	REPS										
	WEIGHT										
	REPS										

NOTES–*(Energy levels, thoughts, adjustments needed.)*

DATE _____

BREAKFAST		MACROS	
		PROTEIN	%
		CARBS	%
		FAT	%
		CALORIES	

LUNCH		MACROS	
		PROTEIN	%
		CARBS	%
		FAT	%
		CALORIES	

DINNER		MACROS	
		PROTEIN	%
		CARBS	%
		FAT	%
		CALORIES	

SNACKS		MACROS	
		PROTEIN	%
		CARBS	%
		FAT	%
		CALORIES	

SUPPLEMENTS		TOTAL MACROS	
		PROTEIN	%
		CARBS	%
		FAT	%
		CALORIES	

NOTES

WATER (12 OZ)

DATE _____

EXERCISE	SETS	1	2	3	4	5	6	7	8	9	10
	WEIGHT										
	REPS										
	WEIGHT										
	REPS										
	WEIGHT										
	REPS										
	WEIGHT										
	REPS										
	WEIGHT										
	REPS										
	WEIGHT										
	REPS										
	WEIGHT										
	REPS										
	WEIGHT										
	REPS										
	WEIGHT										
	REPS										

NOTES–(Energy levels, thoughts, adjustments needed.)

DATE _____

BREAKFAST

MACROS		
PROTEIN		%
CARBS		%
FAT		%
CALORIES		

LUNCH

MACROS		
PROTEIN		%
CARBS		%
FAT		%
CALORIES		

DINNER

MACROS		
PROTEIN		%
CARBS		%
FAT		%
CALORIES		

SNACKS

MACROS		
PROTEIN		%
CARBS		%
FAT		%
CALORIES		

SUPPLEMENTS

TOTAL MACROS		
PROTEIN		%
CARBS		%
FAT		%
CALORIES		

NOTES

WATER (12 OZ)

DATE _____

EXERCISE	SETS	1	2	3	4	5	6	7	8	9	10
	WEIGHT										
	REPS										
	WEIGHT										
	REPS										
	WEIGHT										
	REPS										
	WEIGHT										
	REPS										
	WEIGHT										
	REPS										
	WEIGHT										
	REPS										
	WEIGHT										
	REPS										
	WEIGHT										
	REPS										
	WEIGHT										
	REPS										

NOTES–(Energy levels, thoughts, adjustments needed.)

DATE _____

BREAKFAST

MACROS	
PROTEIN	%
CARBS	%
FAT	%
CALORIES	

LUNCH

MACROS	
PROTEIN	%
CARBS	%
FAT	%
CALORIES	

DINNER

MACROS	
PROTEIN	%
CARBS	%
FAT	%
CALORIES	

SNACKS

MACROS	
PROTEIN	%
CARBS	%
FAT	%
CALORIES	

SUPPLEMENTS

TOTAL MACROS	
PROTEIN	%
CARBS	%
FAT	%
CALORIES	

NOTES

WATER (12 OZ)

DATE _____

EXERCISE	SETS	1	2	3	4	5	6	7	8	9	10
	WEIGHT										
	REPS										
	WEIGHT										
	REPS										
	WEIGHT										
	REPS										
	WEIGHT										
	REPS										
	WEIGHT										
	REPS										
	WEIGHT										
	REPS										
	WEIGHT										
	REPS										
	WEIGHT										
	REPS										
	WEIGHT										
	REPS										

NOTES–*(Energy levels, thoughts, adjustments needed.)*

DATE _____

BREAKFAST

MACROS	
PROTEIN	%
CARBS	%
FAT	%
CALORIES	

LUNCH

MACROS	
PROTEIN	%
CARBS	%
FAT	%
CALORIES	

DINNER

MACROS	
PROTEIN	%
CARBS	%
FAT	%
CALORIES	

SNACKS

MACROS	
PROTEIN	%
CARBS	%
FAT	%
CALORIES	

SUPPLEMENTS

TOTAL MACROS	
PROTEIN	%
CARBS	%
FAT	%
CALORIES	

NOTES

WATER (12 OZ)

DATE _____

EXERCISE	SETS	1	2	3	4	5	6	7	8	9	10
	WEIGHT										
	REPS										
	WEIGHT										
	REPS										
	WEIGHT										
	REPS										
	WEIGHT										
	REPS										
	WEIGHT										
	REPS										
	WEIGHT										
	REPS										
	WEIGHT										
	REPS										
	WEIGHT										
	REPS										
	WEIGHT										
	REPS										

NOTES–(Energy levels, thoughts, adjustments needed.)

DATE _____

BREAKFAST

MACROS	
PROTEIN	%
CARBS	%
FAT	%
CALORIES	

LUNCH

MACROS	
PROTEIN	%
CARBS	%
FAT	%
CALORIES	

DINNER

MACROS	
PROTEIN	%
CARBS	%
FAT	%
CALORIES	

SNACKS

MACROS	
PROTEIN	%
CARBS	%
FAT	%
CALORIES	

SUPPLEMENTS

TOTAL MACROS	
PROTEIN	%
CARBS	%
FAT	%
CALORIES	

NOTES

WATER (12 OZ)

DATE _____

EXERCISE	SETS	1	2	3	4	5	6	7	8	9	10
	WEIGHT										
	REPS										
	WEIGHT										
	REPS										
	WEIGHT										
	REPS										
	WEIGHT										
	REPS										
	WEIGHT										
	REPS										
	WEIGHT										
	REPS										
	WEIGHT										
	REPS										
	WEIGHT										
	REPS										
	WEIGHT										
	REPS										

NOTES–*(Energy levels, thoughts, adjustments needed.)*

DATE _____

BREAKFAST		MACROS	
		PROTEIN	%
		CARBS	%
		FAT	%
		CALORIES	

LUNCH		MACROS	
		PROTEIN	%
		CARBS	%
		FAT	%
		CALORIES	

DINNER		MACROS	
		PROTEIN	%
		CARBS	%
		FAT	%
		CALORIES	

SNACKS		MACROS	
		PROTEIN	%
		CARBS	%
		FAT	%
		CALORIES	

SUPPLEMENTS		TOTAL MACROS	
		PROTEIN	%
		CARBS	%
		FAT	%
		CALORIES	

NOTES

WATER (12 OZ)

DATE _____

EXERCISE	SETS	1	2	3	4	5	6	7	8	9	10
	WEIGHT										
	REPS										
	WEIGHT										
	REPS										
	WEIGHT										
	REPS										
	WEIGHT										
	REPS										
	WEIGHT										
	REPS										
	WEIGHT										
	REPS										
	WEIGHT										
	REPS										
	WEIGHT										
	REPS										
	WEIGHT										
	REPS										

NOTES–*(Energy levels, thoughts, adjustments needed.)*

DATE _____

BREAKFAST		MACROS	
		PROTEIN	%
		CARBS	%
		FAT	%
		CALORIES	

LUNCH		MACROS	
		PROTEIN	%
		CARBS	%
		FAT	%
		CALORIES	

DINNER		MACROS	
		PROTEIN	%
		CARBS	%
		FAT	%
		CALORIES	

SNACKS		MACROS	
		PROTEIN	%
		CARBS	%
		FAT	%
		CALORIES	

SUPPLEMENTS		TOTAL MACROS	
		PROTEIN	%
		CARBS	%
		FAT	%
		CALORIES	

NOTES

WATER (12 OZ)

DATE _____

EXERCISE	SETS	1	2	3	4	5	6	7	8	9	10
	WEIGHT										
	REPS										
	WEIGHT										
	REPS										
	WEIGHT										
	REPS										
	WEIGHT										
	REPS										
	WEIGHT										
	REPS										
	WEIGHT										
	REPS										
	WEIGHT										
	REPS										
	WEIGHT										
	REPS										
	WEIGHT										
	REPS										

NOTES–*(Energy levels, thoughts, adjustments needed.)*

DATE _____

<table>
<tr><td rowspan="5">BREAKFAST</td><td colspan="3">MACROS</td></tr>
<tr><td>PROTEIN</td><td></td><td>%</td></tr>
<tr><td>CARBS</td><td></td><td>%</td></tr>
<tr><td>FAT</td><td></td><td>%</td></tr>
<tr><td>**CALORIES**</td><td></td><td></td></tr>
</table>

<table>
<tr><td rowspan="5">LUNCH</td><td colspan="3">MACROS</td></tr>
<tr><td>PROTEIN</td><td></td><td>%</td></tr>
<tr><td>CARBS</td><td></td><td>%</td></tr>
<tr><td>FAT</td><td></td><td>%</td></tr>
<tr><td>CALORIES</td><td></td><td></td></tr>
</table>

<table>
<tr><td rowspan="5">DINNER</td><td colspan="3">MACROS</td></tr>
<tr><td>PROTEIN</td><td></td><td>%</td></tr>
<tr><td>CARBS</td><td></td><td>%</td></tr>
<tr><td>FAT</td><td></td><td>%</td></tr>
<tr><td>CALORIES</td><td></td><td></td></tr>
</table>

<table>
<tr><td rowspan="5">SNACKS</td><td colspan="3">MACROS</td></tr>
<tr><td>PROTEIN</td><td></td><td>%</td></tr>
<tr><td>CARBS</td><td></td><td>%</td></tr>
<tr><td>FAT</td><td></td><td>%</td></tr>
<tr><td>CALORIES</td><td></td><td></td></tr>
</table>

<table>
<tr><td rowspan="5">SUPPLEMENTS</td><td colspan="3">TOTAL MACROS</td></tr>
<tr><td>PROTEIN</td><td></td><td>%</td></tr>
<tr><td>CARBS</td><td></td><td>%</td></tr>
<tr><td>FAT</td><td></td><td>%</td></tr>
<tr><td>CALORIES</td><td></td><td></td></tr>
</table>

NOTES

WATER (12 OZ)

DATE _____

EXERCISE	SETS	1	2	3	4	5	6	7	8	9	10
	WEIGHT										
	REPS										
	WEIGHT										
	REPS										
	WEIGHT										
	REPS										
	WEIGHT										
	REPS										
	WEIGHT										
	REPS										
	WEIGHT										
	REPS										
	WEIGHT										
	REPS										
	WEIGHT										
	REPS										
	WEIGHT										
	REPS										

NOTES–(Energy levels, thoughts, adjustments needed.)

DATE _____

BREAKFAST		MACROS	
		PROTEIN	%
		CARBS	%
		FAT	%
		CALORIES	

LUNCH		MACROS	
		PROTEIN	%
		CARBS	%
		FAT	%
		CALORIES	

DINNER		MACROS	
		PROTEIN	%
		CARBS	%
		FAT	%
		CALORIES	

SNACKS		MACROS	
		PROTEIN	%
		CARBS	%
		FAT	%
		CALORIES	

SUPPLEMENTS		TOTAL MACROS	
		PROTEIN	%
		CARBS	%
		FAT	%
		CALORIES	

NOTES

WATER (12 OZ)

DATE _____

EXERCISE	SETS	1	2	3	4	5	6	7	8	9	10
	WEIGHT										
	REPS										
	WEIGHT										
	REPS										
	WEIGHT										
	REPS										
	WEIGHT										
	REPS										
	WEIGHT										
	REPS										
	WEIGHT										
	REPS										
	WEIGHT										
	REPS										
	WEIGHT										
	REPS										
	WEIGHT										
	REPS										

NOTES–(Energy levels, thoughts, adjustments needed.)

DATE _____

BREAKFAST	

MACROS	
PROTEIN	%
CARBS	%
FAT	%
CALORIES	

LUNCH	

MACROS	
PROTEIN	%
CARBS	%
FAT	%
CALORIES	

DINNER	

MACROS	
PROTEIN	%
CARBS	%
FAT	%
CALORIES	

SNACKS	

MACROS	
PROTEIN	%
CARBS	%
FAT	%
CALORIES	

SUPPLEMENTS	

TOTAL MACROS	
PROTEIN	%
CARBS	%
FAT	%
CALORIES	

NOTES

WATER (12 OZ)

DATE _____

EXERCISE	SETS	1	2	3	4	5	6	7	8	9	10
	WEIGHT										
	REPS										
	WEIGHT										
	REPS										
	WEIGHT										
	REPS										
	WEIGHT										
	REPS										
	WEIGHT										
	REPS										
	WEIGHT										
	REPS										
	WEIGHT										
	REPS										
	WEIGHT										
	REPS										
	WEIGHT										
	REPS										

NOTES–*(Energy levels, thoughts, adjustments needed.)*

DATE _____

BREAKFAST		MACROS	
		PROTEIN	%
		CARBS	%
		FAT	%
		CALORIES	

LUNCH		MACROS	
		PROTEIN	%
		CARBS	%
		FAT	%
		CALORIES	

DINNER		MACROS	
		PROTEIN	%
		CARBS	%
		FAT	%
		CALORIES	

SNACKS		MACROS	
		PROTEIN	%
		CARBS	%
		FAT	%
		CALORIES	

SUPPLEMENTS		TOTAL MACROS	
		PROTEIN	%
		CARBS	%
		FAT	%
		CALORIES	

NOTES

WATER (12 OZ)

DATE _____

EXERCISE	SETS	1	2	3	4	5	6	7	8	9	10
	WEIGHT										
	REPS										
	WEIGHT										
	REPS										
	WEIGHT										
	REPS										
	WEIGHT										
	REPS										
	WEIGHT										
	REPS										
	WEIGHT										
	REPS										
	WEIGHT										
	REPS										
	WEIGHT										
	REPS										
	WEIGHT										
	REPS										

NOTES–*(Energy levels, thoughts, adjustments needed.)*

DATE _____

BREAKFAST

MACROS		
PROTEIN		%
CARBS		%
FAT		%
CALORIES		

LUNCH

MACROS		
PROTEIN		%
CARBS		%
FAT		%
CALORIES		

DINNER

MACROS		
PROTEIN		%
CARBS		%
FAT		%
CALORIES		

SNACKS

MACROS		
PROTEIN		%
CARBS		%
FAT		%
CALORIES		

SUPPLEMENTS

TOTAL MACROS		
PROTEIN		%
CARBS		%
FAT		%
CALORIES		

NOTES

WATER (12 OZ)

DATE _____

EXERCISE	SETS	1	2	3	4	5	6	7	8	9	10
	WEIGHT										
	REPS										
	WEIGHT										
	REPS										
	WEIGHT										
	REPS										
	WEIGHT										
	REPS										
	WEIGHT										
	REPS										
	WEIGHT										
	REPS										
	WEIGHT										
	REPS										
	WEIGHT										
	REPS										
	WEIGHT										
	REPS										

NOTES–(Energy levels, thoughts, adjustments needed.)

DATE _____

BREAKFAST		MACROS	
		PROTEIN	%
		CARBS	%
		FAT	%
		CALORIES	

LUNCH		MACROS	
		PROTEIN	%
		CARBS	%
		FAT	%
		CALORIES	

DINNER		MACROS	
		PROTEIN	%
		CARBS	%
		FAT	%
		CALORIES	

SNACKS		MACROS	
		PROTEIN	%
		CARBS	%
		FAT	%
		CALORIES	

SUPPLEMENTS		TOTAL MACROS	
		PROTEIN	%
		CARBS	%
		FAT	%
		CALORIES	

NOTES

WATER (12 OZ)

DATE _____

EXERCISE	SETS	1	2	3	4	5	6	7	8	9	10
	WEIGHT										
	REPS										
	WEIGHT										
	REPS										
	WEIGHT										
	REPS										
	WEIGHT										
	REPS										
	WEIGHT										
	REPS										
	WEIGHT										
	REPS										
	WEIGHT										
	REPS										
	WEIGHT										
	REPS										
	WEIGHT										
	REPS										

NOTES–(Energy levels, thoughts, adjustments needed.)

DATE _____

BREAKFAST

MACROS	
PROTEIN	%
CARBS	%
FAT	%
CALORIES	

LUNCH

MACROS	
PROTEIN	%
CARBS	%
FAT	%
CALORIES	

DINNER

MACROS	
PROTEIN	%
CARBS	%
FAT	%
CALORIES	

SNACKS

MACROS	
PROTEIN	%
CARBS	%
FAT	%
CALORIES	

SUPPLEMENTS

TOTAL MACROS	
PROTEIN	%
CARBS	%
FAT	%
CALORIES	

NOTES

WATER (12 OZ)

DATE _____

EXERCISE	SETS	1	2	3	4	5	6	7	8	9	10
	WEIGHT										
	REPS										
	WEIGHT										
	REPS										
	WEIGHT										
	REPS										
	WEIGHT										
	REPS										
	WEIGHT										
	REPS										
	WEIGHT										
	REPS										
	WEIGHT										
	REPS										
	WEIGHT										
	REPS										
	WEIGHT										
	REPS										

NOTES–(Energy levels, thoughts, adjustments needed.)

DATE _____

BREAKFAST

MACROS	
PROTEIN	%
CARBS	%
FAT	%
CALORIES	

LUNCH

MACROS	
PROTEIN	%
CARBS	%
FAT	%
CALORIES	

DINNER

MACROS	
PROTEIN	%
CARBS	%
FAT	%
CALORIES	

SNACKS

MACROS	
PROTEIN	%
CARBS	%
FAT	%
CALORIES	

SUPPLEMENTS

TOTAL MACROS	
PROTEIN	%
CARBS	%
FAT	%
CALORIES	

NOTES

WATER (12 OZ)

DATE _____

EXERCISE	SETS	1	2	3	4	5	6	7	8	9	10
	WEIGHT										
	REPS										
	WEIGHT										
	REPS										
	WEIGHT										
	REPS										
	WEIGHT										
	REPS										
	WEIGHT										
	REPS										
	WEIGHT										
	REPS										
	WEIGHT										
	REPS										
	WEIGHT										
	REPS										
	WEIGHT										
	REPS										

NOTES–(Energy levels, thoughts, adjustments needed.)

DATE _____

BREAKFAST

MACROS		
PROTEIN		%
CARBS		%
FAT		%
CALORIES		

LUNCH

MACROS		
PROTEIN		%
CARBS		%
FAT		%
CALORIES		

DINNER

MACROS		
PROTEIN		%
CARBS		%
FAT		%
CALORIES		

SNACKS

MACROS		
PROTEIN		%
CARBS		%
FAT		%
CALORIES		

SUPPLEMENTS

TOTAL MACROS		
PROTEIN		%
CARBS		%
FAT		%
CALORIES		

NOTES

WATER (12 OZ)

DATE _____

EXERCISE	SETS	1	2	3	4	5	6	7	8	9	10
	WEIGHT										
	REPS										
	WEIGHT										
	REPS										
	WEIGHT										
	REPS										
	WEIGHT										
	REPS										
	WEIGHT										
	REPS										
	WEIGHT										
	REPS										
	WEIGHT										
	REPS										
	WEIGHT										
	REPS										
	WEIGHT										
	REPS										

NOTES–(Energy levels, thoughts, adjustments needed.)

DATE _____

BREAKFAST

MACROS	
PROTEIN	%
CARBS	%
FAT	%
CALORIES	

LUNCH

MACROS	
PROTEIN	%
CARBS	%
FAT	%
CALORIES	

DINNER

MACROS	
PROTEIN	%
CARBS	%
FAT	%
CALORIES	

SNACKS

MACROS	
PROTEIN	%
CARBS	%
FAT	%
CALORIES	

SUPPLEMENTS

TOTAL MACROS	
PROTEIN	%
CARBS	%
FAT	%
CALORIES	

NOTES

WATER (12 OZ)

DATE _____

EXERCISE	SETS	1	2	3	4	5	6	7	8	9	10
	WEIGHT										
	REPS										
	WEIGHT										
	REPS										
	WEIGHT										
	REPS										
	WEIGHT										
	REPS										
	WEIGHT										
	REPS										
	WEIGHT										
	REPS										
	WEIGHT										
	REPS										
	WEIGHT										
	REPS										
	WEIGHT										
	REPS										

NOTES–*(Energy levels, thoughts, adjustments needed.)*

DATE _____

BREAKFAST

MACROS	
PROTEIN	%
CARBS	%
FAT	%
CALORIES	

LUNCH

MACROS	
PROTEIN	%
CARBS	%
FAT	%
CALORIES	

DINNER

MACROS	
PROTEIN	%
CARBS	%
FAT	%
CALORIES	

SNACKS

MACROS	
PROTEIN	%
CARBS	%
FAT	%
CALORIES	

SUPPLEMENTS

TOTAL MACROS	
PROTEIN	%
CARBS	%
FAT	%
CALORIES	

NOTES

WATER (12 OZ)

DATE _____

EXERCISE	SETS	1	2	3	4	5	6	7	8	9	10
	WEIGHT										
	REPS										
	WEIGHT										
	REPS										
	WEIGHT										
	REPS										
	WEIGHT										
	REPS										
	WEIGHT										
	REPS										
	WEIGHT										
	REPS										
	WEIGHT										
	REPS										
	WEIGHT										
	REPS										
	WEIGHT										
	REPS										

NOTES–*(Energy levels, thoughts, adjustments needed.)*

DATE _____

BREAKFAST		MACROS	
	PROTEIN		%
	CARBS		%
	FAT		%
	CALORIES		

LUNCH		MACROS	
	PROTEIN		%
	CARBS		%
	FAT		%
	CALORIES		

DINNER		MACROS	
	PROTEIN		%
	CARBS		%
	FAT		%
	CALORIES		

SNACKS		MACROS	
	PROTEIN		%
	CARBS		%
	FAT		%
	CALORIES		

SUPPLEMENTS		TOTAL MACROS	
	PROTEIN		%
	CARBS		%
	FAT		%
	CALORIES		

NOTES

WATER (12 OZ)

DATE _____

EXERCISE	SETS	1	2	3	4	5	6	7	8	9	10
	WEIGHT										
	REPS										
	WEIGHT										
	REPS										
	WEIGHT										
	REPS										
	WEIGHT										
	REPS										
	WEIGHT										
	REPS										
	WEIGHT										
	REPS										
	WEIGHT										
	REPS										
	WEIGHT										
	REPS										
	WEIGHT										
	REPS										

NOTES–(Energy levels, thoughts, adjustments needed.)

DATE _____

BREAKFAST		MACROS	
		PROTEIN	%
		CARBS	%
		FAT	%
		CALORIES	

LUNCH		MACROS	
		PROTEIN	%
		CARBS	%
		FAT	%
		CALORIES	

DINNER		MACROS	
		PROTEIN	%
		CARBS	%
		FAT	%
		CALORIES	

SNACKS		MACROS	
		PROTEIN	%
		CARBS	%
		FAT	%
		CALORIES	

SUPPLEMENTS		TOTAL MACROS	
		PROTEIN	%
		CARBS	%
		FAT	%
		CALORIES	

NOTES

WATER (12 OZ)

DATE _____

EXERCISE	SETS	1	2	3	4	5	6	7	8	9	10
	WEIGHT										
	REPS										
	WEIGHT										
	REPS										
	WEIGHT										
	REPS										
	WEIGHT										
	REPS										
	WEIGHT										
	REPS										
	WEIGHT										
	REPS										
	WEIGHT										
	REPS										
	WEIGHT										
	REPS										
	WEIGHT										
	REPS										

NOTES–(Energy levels, thoughts, adjustments needed.)

DATE _____

BREAKFAST

MACROS	
PROTEIN	%
CARBS	%
FAT	%
CALORIES	

LUNCH

MACROS	
PROTEIN	%
CARBS	%
FAT	%
CALORIES	

DINNER

MACROS	
PROTEIN	%
CARBS	%
FAT	%
CALORIES	

SNACKS

MACROS	
PROTEIN	%
CARBS	%
FAT	%
CALORIES	

SUPPLEMENTS

TOTAL MACROS	
PROTEIN	%
CARBS	%
FAT	%
CALORIES	

NOTES

WATER (12 OZ)

DATE _____

EXERCISE	SETS	1	2	3	4	5	6	7	8	9	10
	WEIGHT										
	REPS										
	WEIGHT										
	REPS										
	WEIGHT										
	REPS										
	WEIGHT										
	REPS										
	WEIGHT										
	REPS										
	WEIGHT										
	REPS										
	WEIGHT										
	REPS										
	WEIGHT										
	REPS										
	WEIGHT										
	REPS										

NOTES–*(Energy levels, thoughts, adjustments needed.)*

DATE _____

BREAKFAST

MACROS		
PROTEIN		%
CARBS		%
FAT		%
CALORIES		

LUNCH

MACROS		
PROTEIN		%
CARBS		%
FAT		%
CALORIES		

DINNER

MACROS		
PROTEIN		%
CARBS		%
FAT		%
CALORIES		

SNACKS

MACROS		
PROTEIN		%
CARBS		%
FAT		%
CALORIES		

SUPPLEMENTS

TOTAL MACROS		
PROTEIN		%
CARBS		%
FAT		%
CALORIES		

NOTES

WATER (12 OZ)

DATE _____

EXERCISE	SETS	1	2	3	4	5	6	7	8	9	10
	WEIGHT										
	REPS										
	WEIGHT										
	REPS										
	WEIGHT										
	REPS										
	WEIGHT										
	REPS										
	WEIGHT										
	REPS										
	WEIGHT										
	REPS										
	WEIGHT										
	REPS										
	WEIGHT										
	REPS										
	WEIGHT										
	REPS										

NOTES–(Energy levels, thoughts, adjustments needed.)

DATE _____

BREAKFAST

MACROS		
PROTEIN		%
CARBS		%
FAT		%
CALORIES		

LUNCH

MACROS		
PROTEIN		%
CARBS		%
FAT		%
CALORIES		

DINNER

MACROS		
PROTEIN		%
CARBS		%
FAT		%
CALORIES		

SNACKS

MACROS		
PROTEIN		%
CARBS		%
FAT		%
CALORIES		

SUPPLEMENTS

TOTAL MACROS		
PROTEIN		%
CARBS		%
FAT		%
CALORIES		

NOTES

WATER (12 OZ)

DATE _____

EXERCISE	SETS	1	2	3	4	5	6	7	8	9	10
	WEIGHT										
	REPS										
	WEIGHT										
	REPS										
	WEIGHT										
	REPS										
	WEIGHT										
	REPS										
	WEIGHT										
	REPS										
	WEIGHT										
	REPS										
	WEIGHT										
	REPS										
	WEIGHT										
	REPS										
	WEIGHT										
	REPS										

NOTES–(Energy levels, thoughts, adjustments needed.)

DATE _____

BREAKFAST

MACROS		
PROTEIN		%
CARBS		%
FAT		%
CALORIES		

LUNCH

MACROS		
PROTEIN		%
CARBS		%
FAT		%
CALORIES		

DINNER

MACROS		
PROTEIN		%
CARBS		%
FAT		%
CALORIES		

SNACKS

MACROS		
PROTEIN		%
CARBS		%
FAT		%
CALORIES		

SUPPLEMENTS

TOTAL MACROS		
PROTEIN		%
CARBS		%
FAT		%
CALORIES		

NOTES

WATER (12 OZ)

DATE _____

EXERCISE	SETS	1	2	3	4	5	6	7	8	9	10
	WEIGHT										
	REPS										
	WEIGHT										
	REPS										
	WEIGHT										
	REPS										
	WEIGHT										
	REPS										
	WEIGHT										
	REPS										
	WEIGHT										
	REPS										
	WEIGHT										
	REPS										
	WEIGHT										
	REPS										
	WEIGHT										
	REPS										

NOTES–(Energy levels, thoughts, adjustments needed.)

DATE _____

BREAKFAST

MACROS	
PROTEIN	%
CARBS	%
FAT	%
CALORIES	

LUNCH

MACROS	
PROTEIN	%
CARBS	%
FAT	%
CALORIES	

DINNER

MACROS	
PROTEIN	%
CARBS	%
FAT	%
CALORIES	

SNACKS

MACROS	
PROTEIN	%
CARBS	%
FAT	%
CALORIES	

SUPPLEMENTS

TOTAL MACROS	
PROTEIN	%
CARBS	%
FAT	%
CALORIES	

NOTES

WATER (12 OZ)

DATE _____

EXERCISE	SETS	1	2	3	4	5	6	7	8	9	10
	WEIGHT										
	REPS										
	WEIGHT										
	REPS										
	WEIGHT										
	REPS										
	WEIGHT										
	REPS										
	WEIGHT										
	REPS										
	WEIGHT										
	REPS										
	WEIGHT										
	REPS										
	WEIGHT										
	REPS										
	WEIGHT										
	REPS										

NOTES–*(Energy levels, thoughts, adjustments needed.)*

DATE _____

BREAKFAST		MACROS	
		PROTEIN	%
		CARBS	%
		FAT	%
		CALORIES	

LUNCH		MACROS	
		PROTEIN	%
		CARBS	%
		FAT	%
		CALORIES	

DINNER		MACROS	
		PROTEIN	%
		CARBS	%
		FAT	%
		CALORIES	

SNACKS		MACROS	
		PROTEIN	%
		CARBS	%
		FAT	%
		CALORIES	

SUPPLEMENTS		TOTAL MACROS	
		PROTEIN	%
		CARBS	%
		FAT	%
		CALORIES	

NOTES

WATER (12 OZ)

DATE _____

EXERCISE	SETS	1	2	3	4	5	6	7	8	9	10
	WEIGHT										
	REPS										
	WEIGHT										
	REPS										
	WEIGHT										
	REPS										
	WEIGHT										
	REPS										
	WEIGHT										
	REPS										
	WEIGHT										
	REPS										
	WEIGHT										
	REPS										
	WEIGHT										
	REPS										
	WEIGHT										
	REPS										

NOTES–(Energy levels, thoughts, adjustments needed.)

DATE _____

BREAKFAST		MACROS	
		PROTEIN	%
		CARBS	%
		FAT	%
		CALORIES	

LUNCH		MACROS	
		PROTEIN	%
		CARBS	%
		FAT	%
		CALORIES	

DINNER		MACROS	
		PROTEIN	%
		CARBS	%
		FAT	%
		CALORIES	

SNACKS		MACROS	
		PROTEIN	%
		CARBS	%
		FAT	%
		CALORIES	

SUPPLEMENTS		TOTAL MACROS	
		PROTEIN	%
		CARBS	%
		FAT	%
		CALORIES	

NOTES

WATER (12 OZ)

DATE _____

EXERCISE	SETS	1	2	3	4	5	6	7	8	9	10
	WEIGHT										
	REPS										
	WEIGHT										
	REPS										
	WEIGHT										
	REPS										
	WEIGHT										
	REPS										
	WEIGHT										
	REPS										
	WEIGHT										
	REPS										
	WEIGHT										
	REPS										
	WEIGHT										
	REPS										
	WEIGHT										
	REPS										

NOTES–*(Energy levels, thoughts, adjustments needed.)*

DATE _____

BREAKFAST

MACROS	
PROTEIN	%
CARBS	%
FAT	%
CALORIES	

LUNCH

MACROS	
PROTEIN	%
CARBS	%
FAT	%
CALORIES	

DINNER

MACROS	
PROTEIN	%
CARBS	%
FAT	%
CALORIES	

SNACKS

MACROS	
PROTEIN	%
CARBS	%
FAT	%
CALORIES	

SUPPLEMENTS

TOTAL MACROS	
PROTEIN	%
CARBS	%
FAT	%
CALORIES	

NOTES

WATER (12 OZ)

DATE _____

EXERCISE	SETS	1	2	3	4	5	6	7	8	9	10
	WEIGHT										
	REPS										
	WEIGHT										
	REPS										
	WEIGHT										
	REPS										
	WEIGHT										
	REPS										
	WEIGHT										
	REPS										
	WEIGHT										
	REPS										
	WEIGHT										
	REPS										
	WEIGHT										
	REPS										
	WEIGHT										
	REPS										

NOTES–(Energy levels, thoughts, adjustments needed.)

DATE _____

BREAKFAST		MACROS	
		PROTEIN	%
		CARBS	%
		FAT	%
		CALORIES	

LUNCH		MACROS	
		PROTEIN	%
		CARBS	%
		FAT	%
		CALORIES	

DINNER		MACROS	
		PROTEIN	%
		CARBS	%
		FAT	%
		CALORIES	

SNACKS		MACROS	
		PROTEIN	%
		CARBS	%
		FAT	%
		CALORIES	

SUPPLEMENTS		TOTAL MACROS	
		PROTEIN	%
		CARBS	%
		FAT	%
		CALORIES	

NOTES

WATER (12 OZ)

DATE _____

EXERCISE	SETS	1	2	3	4	5	6	7	8	9	10
	WEIGHT										
	REPS										
	WEIGHT										
	REPS										
	WEIGHT										
	REPS										
	WEIGHT										
	REPS										
	WEIGHT										
	REPS										
	WEIGHT										
	REPS										
	WEIGHT										
	REPS										
	WEIGHT										
	REPS										
	WEIGHT										
	REPS										

NOTES–*(Energy levels, thoughts, adjustments needed.)*

DATE _____

BREAKFAST		MACROS	
		PROTEIN	%
		CARBS	%
		FAT	%
		CALORIES	

LUNCH		MACROS	
		PROTEIN	%
		CARBS	%
		FAT	%
		CALORIES	

DINNER		MACROS	
		PROTEIN	%
		CARBS	%
		FAT	%
		CALORIES	

SNACKS		MACROS	
		PROTEIN	%
		CARBS	%
		FAT	%
		CALORIES	

SUPPLEMENTS		TOTAL MACROS	
		PROTEIN	%
		CARBS	%
		FAT	%
		CALORIES	

NOTES

WATER (12 OZ)

DATE _____

EXERCISE	SETS	1	2	3	4	5	6	7	8	9	10
	WEIGHT										
	REPS										
	WEIGHT										
	REPS										
	WEIGHT										
	REPS										
	WEIGHT										
	REPS										
	WEIGHT										
	REPS										
	WEIGHT										
	REPS										
	WEIGHT										
	REPS										
	WEIGHT										
	REPS										
	WEIGHT										
	REPS										

NOTES–(Energy levels, thoughts, adjustments needed.)

DATE _____

BREAKFAST		MACROS	
		PROTEIN	%
		CARBS	%
		FAT	%
		CALORIES	

LUNCH		MACROS	
		PROTEIN	%
		CARBS	%
		FAT	%
		CALORIES	

DINNER		MACROS	
		PROTEIN	%
		CARBS	%
		FAT	%
		CALORIES	

SNACKS		MACROS	
		PROTEIN	%
		CARBS	%
		FAT	%
		CALORIES	

SUPPLEMENTS		TOTAL MACROS	
		PROTEIN	%
		CARBS	%
		FAT	%
		CALORIES	

NOTES

WATER (12 OZ)

DATE _____

EXERCISE	SETS	1	2	3	4	5	6	7	8	9	10
	WEIGHT										
	REPS										
	WEIGHT										
	REPS										
	WEIGHT										
	REPS										
	WEIGHT										
	REPS										
	WEIGHT										
	REPS										
	WEIGHT										
	REPS										
	WEIGHT										
	REPS										
	WEIGHT										
	REPS										
	WEIGHT										
	REPS										

NOTES–*(Energy levels, thoughts, adjustments needed.)*

DATE _____

BREAKFAST		MACROS	
		PROTEIN	%
		CARBS	%
		FAT	%
		CALORIES	

LUNCH		MACROS	
		PROTEIN	%
		CARBS	%
		FAT	%
		CALORIES	

DINNER		MACROS	
		PROTEIN	%
		CARBS	%
		FAT	%
		CALORIES	

SNACKS		MACROS	
		PROTEIN	%
		CARBS	%
		FAT	%
		CALORIES	

SUPPLEMENTS		TOTAL MACROS	
		PROTEIN	%
		CARBS	%
		FAT	%
		CALORIES	

NOTES

WATER (12 OZ)

DATE _____

EXERCISE	SETS	1	2	3	4	5	6	7	8	9	10
	WEIGHT										
	REPS										
	WEIGHT										
	REPS										
	WEIGHT										
	REPS										
	WEIGHT										
	REPS										
	WEIGHT										
	REPS										
	WEIGHT										
	REPS										
	WEIGHT										
	REPS										
	WEIGHT										
	REPS										
	WEIGHT										
	REPS										

NOTES–(Energy levels, thoughts, adjustments needed.)

DATE _____

BREAKFAST

MACROS	
PROTEIN	%
CARBS	%
FAT	%
CALORIES	

LUNCH

MACROS	
PROTEIN	%
CARBS	%
FAT	%
CALORIES	

DINNER

MACROS	
PROTEIN	%
CARBS	%
FAT	%
CALORIES	

SNACKS

MACROS	
PROTEIN	%
CARBS	%
FAT	%
CALORIES	

SUPPLEMENTS

TOTAL MACROS	
PROTEIN	%
CARBS	%
FAT	%
CALORIES	

NOTES

WATER (12 OZ)

DATE _____

EXERCISE	SETS	1	2	3	4	5	6	7	8	9	10
	WEIGHT										
	REPS										
	WEIGHT										
	REPS										
	WEIGHT										
	REPS										
	WEIGHT										
	REPS										
	WEIGHT										
	REPS										
	WEIGHT										
	REPS										
	WEIGHT										
	REPS										
	WEIGHT										
	REPS										
	WEIGHT										
	REPS										

NOTES–*(Energy levels, thoughts, adjustments needed.)*

DATE _____

BREAKFAST

MACROS	
PROTEIN	%
CARBS	%
FAT	%
CALORIES	

LUNCH

MACROS	
PROTEIN	%
CARBS	%
FAT	%
CALORIES	

DINNER

MACROS	
PROTEIN	%
CARBS	%
FAT	%
CALORIES	

SNACKS

MACROS	
PROTEIN	%
CARBS	%
FAT	%
CALORIES	

SUPPLEMENTS

TOTAL MACROS	
PROTEIN	%
CARBS	%
FAT	%
CALORIES	

NOTES

WATER (12 OZ)

DATE _____

EXERCISE	SETS	1	2	3	4	5	6	7	8	9	10
	WEIGHT										
	REPS										
	WEIGHT										
	REPS										
	WEIGHT										
	REPS										
	WEIGHT										
	REPS										
	WEIGHT										
	REPS										
	WEIGHT										
	REPS										
	WEIGHT										
	REPS										
	WEIGHT										
	REPS										
	WEIGHT										
	REPS										

NOTES–*(Energy levels, thoughts, adjustments needed.)*

DATE _____

BREAKFAST

MACROS	
PROTEIN	%
CARBS	%
FAT	%
CALORIES	

LUNCH

MACROS	
PROTEIN	%
CARBS	%
FAT	%
CALORIES	

DINNER

MACROS	
PROTEIN	%
CARBS	%
FAT	%
CALORIES	

SNACKS

MACROS	
PROTEIN	%
CARBS	%
FAT	%
CALORIES	

SUPPLEMENTS

TOTAL MACROS	
PROTEIN	%
CARBS	%
FAT	%
CALORIES	

NOTES

WATER (12 OZ)

DATE _____

EXERCISE	SETS	1	2	3	4	5	6	7	8	9	10
	WEIGHT										
	REPS										
	WEIGHT										
	REPS										
	WEIGHT										
	REPS										
	WEIGHT										
	REPS										
	WEIGHT										
	REPS										
	WEIGHT										
	REPS										
	WEIGHT										
	REPS										
	WEIGHT										
	REPS										
	WEIGHT										
	REPS										

NOTES–(Energy levels, thoughts, adjustments needed.)

_____
_____
_____
_____
_____
_____
_____
_____
_____

DATE _____

BREAKFAST		MACROS	
		PROTEIN	%
		CARBS	%
		FAT	%
		CALORIES	

LUNCH		MACROS	
		PROTEIN	%
		CARBS	%
		FAT	%
		CALORIES	

DINNER		MACROS	
		PROTEIN	%
		CARBS	%
		FAT	%
		CALORIES	

SNACKS		MACROS	
		PROTEIN	%
		CARBS	%
		FAT	%
		CALORIES	

SUPPLEMENTS		TOTAL MACROS	
		PROTEIN	%
		CARBS	%
		FAT	%
		CALORIES	

NOTES

WATER (12 OZ)

DATE _____

EXERCISE	SETS	1	2	3	4	5	6	7	8	9	10
	WEIGHT										
	REPS										
	WEIGHT										
	REPS										
	WEIGHT										
	REPS										
	WEIGHT										
	REPS										
	WEIGHT										
	REPS										
	WEIGHT										
	REPS										
	WEIGHT										
	REPS										
	WEIGHT										
	REPS										
	WEIGHT										
	REPS										

NOTES–(Energy levels, thoughts, adjustments needed.)

DATE _____

BREAKFAST

MACROS	
PROTEIN	%
CARBS	%
FAT	%
CALORIES	

LUNCH

MACROS	
PROTEIN	%
CARBS	%
FAT	%
CALORIES	

DINNER

MACROS	
PROTEIN	%
CARBS	%
FAT	%
CALORIES	

SNACKS

MACROS	
PROTEIN	%
CARBS	%
FAT	%
CALORIES	

SUPPLEMENTS

TOTAL MACROS	
PROTEIN	%
CARBS	%
FAT	%
CALORIES	

NOTES

WATER (12 OZ)

DATE _____

EXERCISE	SETS	1	2	3	4	5	6	7	8	9	10
	WEIGHT										
	REPS										
	WEIGHT										
	REPS										
	WEIGHT										
	REPS										
	WEIGHT										
	REPS										
	WEIGHT										
	REPS										
	WEIGHT										
	REPS										
	WEIGHT										
	REPS										
	WEIGHT										
	REPS										
	WEIGHT										
	REPS										

NOTES–*(Energy levels, thoughts, adjustments needed.)*

DATE _____

BREAKFAST

MACROS		
PROTEIN		%
CARBS		%
FAT		%
CALORIES		

LUNCH

MACROS		
PROTEIN		%
CARBS		%
FAT		%
CALORIES		

DINNER

MACROS		
PROTEIN		%
CARBS		%
FAT		%
CALORIES		

SNACKS

MACROS		
PROTEIN		%
CARBS		%
FAT		%
CALORIES		

SUPPLEMENTS

TOTAL MACROS		
PROTEIN		%
CARBS		%
FAT		%
CALORIES		

NOTES

WATER (12 OZ)

DATE _____

EXERCISE	SETS	1	2	3	4	5	6	7	8	9	10
	WEIGHT										
	REPS										
	WEIGHT										
	REPS										
	WEIGHT										
	REPS										
	WEIGHT										
	REPS										
	WEIGHT										
	REPS										
	WEIGHT										
	REPS										
	WEIGHT										
	REPS										
	WEIGHT										
	REPS										
	WEIGHT										
	REPS										

NOTES–(Energy levels, thoughts, adjustments needed.)

DATE _____

BREAKFAST

MACROS	
PROTEIN	%
CARBS	%
FAT	%
CALORIES	

LUNCH

MACROS	
PROTEIN	%
CARBS	%
FAT	%
CALORIES	

DINNER

MACROS	
PROTEIN	%
CARBS	%
FAT	%
CALORIES	

SNACKS

MACROS	
PROTEIN	%
CARBS	%
FAT	%
CALORIES	

SUPPLEMENTS

TOTAL MACROS	
PROTEIN	%
CARBS	%
FAT	%
CALORIES	

NOTES

WATER (12 OZ)

www.ingramcontent.com/pod-product-compliance
Lightning Source LLC
Chambersburg PA
CBHW081556280526
45788CB00011B/3489